CW00428719

ISBN-13: 9798648145207
ISBN-10: 1477123456

Cover design by: Art Painter
Library of Congress Control Number: 2018675309
Printed in the United States of America

I dedicate this book to Mick Johnson for his tireless efforts to keep me smiling everyday x

Contents

Chapter 1

Facing the Giant

As we stumbled up the sandy ridge, my jaw dropped and my eyes widened as I looked down towards the beach. I'd never seen so many sunbathers of this sort, and the wind chill didn't seem to deter them. They lay there basking in the brilliant sunshine as far as the eye could see.

I had to catch my breath, the cold cut through me, and my gloves gave little protection as I fumbled to take good photos. February always seemed to be a harsh month.

Seeing them in the wild like this was so moving and I edged closer to them a little shuffle at a time. There were large pups that soon would be independent scattered about, and some older seals as if on guard duty while the others could just warm up in the sun or splash about in the sea close to the beach. It seemed ideal conditions for them, but we stood there shivering.

The sound of the sea, that unmistakable smell, walking along the beach bare foot with the waves lapping my toes, collecting stones and shells. Fish and chips always tasted better there.

To swim in the sea on a hot day, or even brave a paddle when it wasn't so hot. Sitting on the sand running it through my fingers.

I dreamt of living by the sea with time on my hands for long beach walks. Fresh fish all the time, Mick would cook me fish suppers and we would love every minute.

This was the first time we'd encountered the seals there, but it wouldn't be the last. 2018 had started well and like any other year, Mick and I were focusing on spending as much time at the seaside as possible.

Another cold February back in 2012, it was so bad I had to take a taxi to Mick's house or I would've been a block of ice by the time I got there. We were going out to dinner to an Indian restaurant and Mick's house-mate offered to give us a lift into town. She kindly dropped us fairly close, but even that short walk to the pub was painful, it was cutting through us as we huddled together almost running. Even the pre-dinner drink we had before braving the elements again didn't warm us up. Finally at the Indian we slowly thawed out with our spicy dinner. That was the night Mick asked me to marry him.

We both had fun gathering items for our fancy dress costumes, as our engagement party had an 80's theme. Both of us were 80's punks for the evening, he with his multi-coloured Mohawk and me with my big blue mullet! "It suit's you!" he said, but I wasn't so sure.

Guests came, drink was drunk, food was consumed, although, I don't remember eating much, a few token nibbles and some kind of yummy chocolate cake Mick handed me. We took our own drinks with us and lets face it, as long as I had my rum and coke, all was well. To mark the occasion I may have had a glass of bubbly or two. I was merry, and Mick was in his element. We shuffled on the dance floor quite a bit and before we knew it, we were dancing our last dance to something that slipped my memory. I just recall dancing in the arms of my fella.

Our wedding followed that same year. A wonderful day with just a few guests. We were transported to the registry office on the majestic Mega Decker! (bus driver's privilege!) Decorated inside with balloons and other paraphernalia, better than a limo! Mick managed to get through the ceremony without making a smart remark, I managed not to cry and we had a nice sit down dinner afterwards. Later we enjoyed more drinks as more guests joined us in the evening to celebrate. We were staying at the hotel and when we finally went to our room, realised we hadn't eaten anything for hours. Mick decided to go foraging around the all night supermarket in his wedding gear, so we had a little midnight feast.

The following day we embarked on our blissful honeymoon at the seaside, of course east coast, the place of many happy memories for us.

Ireland was our choice of holiday in May, it was Mick's first flight ever and he said it was his last. With his eyes shut all the way, he really didn't enjoy that part. My encouragement for him to look out the window was to no avail, but for me, my eyes were wide open. I looked down at the clouds and the tiny landscape below, and a wind farm that looked like little match sticks in the sea.

It was my wish to visit the Giant's Causeway as it had always fascinated me. I suppose I liked the legend behind it, of the two giant's from Ireland and Scotland.

There was the scientific explanation, but where's the fun in that!

Legend has it that in ancient times, a giant call Finn McCool lived on the Antrim coast. Across the sea in Scotland was another giant named Benadonner, who was threatening Ireland. Full of rage Finn threw big chunks of rock into the sea, which formed a causeway for him to take his anger out on Benadonner. However, when Finn saw how much more gigantic Benadonner was he ran back home.

Finn's wife quickly disguised him as a baby, which fooled the Scottish giant, believing that if the baby was that big, his father must be massive. Benadonner hastily retreated, ripping up the causeway as he went, so as Finn would not be able to follow.

The remains of the causeway are still in Ireland and Scotland to this day.

I had a wishing well in the garden, Mick built it for me before we were married. For me it was a symbol of good times. Something to dream of, something to wish for. Not to hide, or try to be someone I wasn't. My internal struggle was real, no matter what it looked like on the outside. Things would change and troubles built up, that was the way of life. I had often wished I were different, not liking parts of my personality. The way I cried, when all I wanted was to be so angry! It was probably my safety valve, but it made me feel weak.

I'd always wished for a large family, since I was a child. My Grandma had seven children, my mum being the second oldest. Turned out that seven was a few too many for me, I had four with my first husband.

Being a mum was something I'd wanted to do well in life. I couldn't be pushy, it wasn't in me to do that. I had tried to instil good values in them while they were young and despite any of my flaws, they all grew up to be nice people. This was my goal for them, as what ever they had achieved in life that was because they had done it themselves, and I would be proud of them. If they hadn't turned out to be nice people, I would've considered that failure on my part, as I considered it my job to give them a moral compass.

We had a perfect day, and we parked up at a pub next to the entrance. The pub allowed us to park for free as long as we went in afterwards for a drink, we got this tip from a local taxi driver. It's then free to walk down to the Giant's Causeway, and in the warm sunshine it was a pleasure.

I enjoyed climbing on the rocks, looking in wonder at the columns and shapes. I sat down and put my feet in the sea, which to my mind is the natural thing to do. It whooshed through the rocks over my feet, and the shock of the icy cold water made me squeal, and I'm sure Mick made a similar noise. We laughed again and again as we watched the video we took.

Video's are quite helpful in capturing the essence of a memory. They must be one of the most important things that the mind can do for a person. Without them I think we are lost, as what is life if it isn't the making of memories.

They can come to you out the blue, the other week I remembered Green Shield Stamps, and how as a little girl I would stick them in books for my dad. This must have been stored away somewhere safe in my mind, ready to be brought out when needed.

I thought of my mind as rooms with corridors, like a house. Some rooms are busy, others dark with the door locked. Some people have ordered minds, tidy and uncluttered, some are just full of ideas. Their minds must be different from mine, maybe with revolving doors.

I'd wondered why my memory was so bad but really it wasn't surprising if I had to sprint down corridors to retrieve them. Some sort of filing system would've been better and I was sure many better functioning people had one. It was apparent though, that I couldn't really help the way my mind worked ... at least it worked!

I could exercise it better, get better at running down the corridors and quicker at getting the right key to unlock the doors but the fact remained my mind was a house and an untidy one at that.

We packed in quite a lot into just a few days, driving across the country to Southern Ireland, visiting a friend and then up to Northern Ireland, staying near the Giant's Causeway. We saw how they made the whiskey at Bushmills, and had a few tasters! I wasn't a great whiskey drinker, but that was quality.

The Irish pub we went to, funnily enough was called the Scotch House, and I liked the barman as he was very liberal with the rum!

The holiday was a welcome distraction from the difficult times that fate had laid out before me. I managed to put it all to the back of my mind and enjoy our time away. After all, it was a waiting game a lot of the time and best to get on with things. Worrying doesn't change the outcome.

I'd called up the doctor to be seen for an urgent appointment, I was nervous, I had seen blood in my pee. Only a small amount, it would have been easy to dismiss it, but I worried it could be kidney problems, as my dad had suffered. I was shaking as I told her, then started blubbering, but it was a relief to talk to the doctor about it. She did a test to see if blood was in my urine, and it was confirmed. I was told it could be an infection but it turned out it wasn't.

When I got the appointment at my local hospital to go and have a cystoscopy, where they look inside the bladder with a camera, I really didn't think they would find anything there, I was convinced it was a problem with my kidneys.

I lay there with the nurse talking to me, distracting me, and all of a sudden I saw on the screen, the inside of my bladder, and there they were ... multiple tumours, the lining of my bladder was covered in these things. The doctor had been making some comments which I forget, but I remember saying to him "so what I see there, isn't normal then?" I had to be sure, I mean I've never seen inside my bladder before, he confirmed that it wasn't normal but they would sort it out for me.

In a daze, I went to the cafe to get a coffee, and I sat and stared at it. I don't know how long I was there, and my mind didn't seem to be able to process what had just happened. The pause button had been pressed. Then it seemed to reboot and questions went around in my head, about what was going to happen to me.

After we flew home, Mick said his ears hurt, another reason not to ever fly again, however, he was happy that he had gone through with it, and Ireland can be reached by sea, after all.

I was booked in to have an operation to remove the tumours (TURBT) and they would then do biopsies. They had to establish if it was indeed as sinister as we suspected.

I had been open from the start with my friends at work and throughout it all my colleagues gave me all the time and support that I needed. Focusing on work was a good way to keep moving on, and cope with all the waiting on appointments and results.

Everything had been going so well for me at the pharmacy, I had finally got the shifts I wanted, the hours I wanted. No late nights, I was in the middle of a course and training to be a dispenser as well and really loving it. All this was about to change, as my health had to take priority.

My consultant was a pleasant and humorous man, When I first saw him he laughed and joked with me, he said I was way too young for his clinic, and what was I doing there.

This time was way more serious and although he tried to assure me that everything would be fine and I would live through this, from the moment he said it was cancer, my mind went numb again. I sat on the edge of my seat, listening to him explaining things, shaking a little and trying to hold back the emotions. I was glad Mick was there.

The word 'cancer' had not been mentioned to me before they did the biopsies, but of course, it was going through my mind quite a bit. No matter what anyone said to me at the time, I still thought I was going to die. However, I felt it best to keep that to myself.

My giant's name was Bladder Cancer.

It was an aggressive type that would return even though they had scraped a lot out during the TURBT, and I was being transferred to Addenbrooke's hospital, Cambridge, as they were more specialised in the treatment of bladder cancer.

Things seemed to get extremely serious, extremely quickly.

Chapter 2

"Bugger My Rags"

A curious expression I remember from my childhood ... it was a favourite saying of my grandad (he was my dad's dad) and it always made me laugh when he said it "well, bugger my rags!!" ... it still makes me smile and chuckle, he was so funny.

John was his name but, some people used to call him Jack ... I don't know why!? He would talk to anyone and he had a superb sense of humour. He could do no wrong in my eyes and I think it was because he would always spend time with me when I was a kid. We played cards, went on bike rides and walks, time seemed slower back then. In fact, I think it was slower, at least it was in my young mind, before it became cluttered and messy.

Grandma and grandad's house, had an outside loo, as a child I'd take the torch and venture out, like camping. In each bedroom was a bucket, for those that didn't want to brave the elements in the middle of the night when the house was locked up.

They also had a real fire, so winter evenings only the front room was hot, and the rest of the house was left freezing. My brother and I thought it was great fun poking it to make things burn, and watching as it consumed everything we threw on it. Grandma had two rugs for the front of the fire, in summer it was an orange one, and in winter when the fire was lit, it was a black one, I think that was sensible. Every now and then, grandad would have to sweep the chimney, and my job was to stand outside and shout when I saw the top of the brush pop out of the chimney.

The memories of those times would come back in later years, when I'd sit outside feeding the fire in the yard with blocks of wood. Staring at it as the flames danced and feeling the warmth and basking in the glow.

Young Nicky didn't have a care in the world, well except my parents divorced and a step dad was on the scene, though I felt like I took that in my stride and the consequence of that was more time at grandma and grandad's where my dad was living.

So, weekends were great up to the age of eleven, this was when my mum died. My world had been shattered, and as you may guess, life changed for me and my brother, and "bugger my rags" doesn't even begin to describe what I felt that night when everything was thrown into disarray.

A mind that was carefree became numb, how else do you defend yourself in this world, I have learned that pain needs to be numbed so that life can carry on, which it does even when you want it to stop so badly.

Time seemed to speed up a bit from then on and my mind de-fogged a bit at a time, but a numb mind will feel the pain eventually.

Addenbrooke's hospital was massive. Once we found somewhere to park the car, we trudged round the grounds and the corridors and eventually found the clinic.

I had visited years ago when my dad was ill, but things had changed dramatically since then. There were all manner of shops and cafes, fast food places, banks and a hairdresser, every thing you wanted really.

We were led by a specialist nurse to a small room and we all waited for the consultant to arrive. He greeted us and perched himself on the examination couch. He was cool, calm and collected, and put us at ease straight away. After quite a lengthy discussion, I was told they wanted to do another investigation (TURBT) themselves.

Again I had to prepare for it, being more worried than I was before. This was a different hospital, different ways, different doctors, and the last one I had was very uncomfortable afterwards to say the least.

Going through procedures for the first time is rather daunting, even when they supposedly tell you what's going to happen, it rarely goes by the book. Like my first CT scan, I had to change into one of those gowns, now I know better, as long a I wasn't wearing metal, normal clothes were OK, forget the faffing about, t-shirt and leggings/jogging bottoms are fine.

It wasn't just a scan, they had to inject a dye substance in through a cannula in my arm. Now this didn't phase me really, it wasn't a problem, but as I lay on the bench the nurse told me that it would most probably feel like I had pee'd myself when the dye goes through my system! I laughed of course, not quite believing it, but low and behold they were right, and I have to tell you when I got up I had to check my hospital gown wasn't wet! I mean in those days, when I needed to go to the toilet, I really needed to go, so I was relieved that all was well.

The first TURBT I had was at my local hospital, Bedford. It was a day surgery, but I had to bring a bag just in case I had to stay overnight. When I woke up after the procedure, I was very sore down below, I had a catheter bag and it just made me feel like I wanted to go to the toilet all the time, even though it was obviously taking care of that for me. Thankfully, after a while they took it away, and I was allowed to go home and rest. It was uncomfortable and I took pain killers, they had done a lot of work removing all that cancer. I was told to drink loads, and had to go to the toilet very frequently.

I had to have bloods taken and scans, and another pre-op appointment with the nurse once the date was set for my second TURBT.

I said to the nurse that I thought my period landed on that date, and would it be ok because I felt rather awkward about it. She said it wouldn't affect the procedure. I was hoping my period would be delayed but alas I had to suck in the embarrassment, and carry on. Knowing the doctors and nurses have seen it all before still doesn't stop those feelings.

Waking up again afterwards, I felt so much better than the last time. I didn't have a catheter in, and it wasn't as sore. The procedure hadn't taken long and I was allowed home to rest again, with the same advice.

To cope in the past I have had very simple ways of conditioning my mind to focus. I find that for my particular type of mind, for me to stay reasonably sane (if that be possible) I have little things which I like to look at that give me a sense of individuality and make me feel good for that moment. I suppose it's a bit like mindfulness, although I was doing it long before it was called that.

Years ago I had a candle lighting ritual, I would light a candle, a little enjoyment came from it and made a task more bearable. Another little pleasure was fish corner, three fish pictures on my wall. I'd look at them and wonder about them, I guess my mind needs these things to get by from day to day. Like a day dream, it does us good for our minds to wander into nonsense sometimes.

We had tropical fish, they were relaxing to watch and lovely and colourful but before I met Mick, I was a bit traumatised when one of my fish (a rather large loach) committed suicide one evening while I was changing the water. Out it flipped right down the back of the aquarium where I couldn't get it! I could hear it flipping about but couldn't save him! Obviously after a while he was dead so I thought I would try to get him out from behind in the morning, only to walk in the next day to see the dog having a great game of flip the fish! At the time I was horrified and truly upset, I now see the amusing side.

The biggest coping mechanism is my sense of humour, without it I would have died from the stress, worry and fear – the cancer wouldn't have got a look in!

Back at the clinic I was waiting to hear the results of the second TURBT. I had already been given an outline as to possible treatments for my cancer.

My choices to think about were:

- Treatment with BCG (a type of immunotherapy drug) put straight into the bladder to possibly stunt any re-growth of the cancer, there would be several doses over a period of time, followed by a Cystoscopy at regular intervals.

- Removal of bladder and formation of an ileal conduit and stoma, basically a bag for life.

- Removal of bladder and formation of a neobladder (a new bladder made out of intestine) this would be in the same place as the old bladder, but learning how to use it would be a difficult process as it wouldn't have the same feeling as a normal bladder.

Lots of thought went into deciding what to do, and I had already decided to go with surgery, and the neobladder was my first choice.

As my cancer was aggressive, I didn't want to keep my bladder and risk it spreading. For me it was a fairly easy choice, for me it was live without my bladder or die with it. I had looked at all the statistics, I did my research, and I was 49 years old, I wanted to live a lot longer, so my mind was made up.

When it came to the results, I was shocked again when the consultant told me more cancer was found, in my urethra this time, a different type again, and still aggressive.

Every thing was up in the air again! he told me BCG wouldn't be effective anyway because of where the cancer was, and also I couldn't have the neobladder because my urethra would have to be removed along with my bladder so peeing in the normal way was out of the question!

I think my grandad's phrase..."*bugger my rags!*" comes into play here.

Remaining calm but in a little voice, I said, "so it has to be a bag then?" to which he replied with a little sideways smile, "well, not necessarily, there is a different way".

Gaining my interest, he went on to explain that they could build me a new bladder (internal reservoir/pouch) from part of my intestine, and use my appendix to make a tube, which when in place I would be able put a catheter into my tummy button and the urine would come out! I would be able to pee standing up!

They said it was called a mitrofanoff.

I had never heard of this before, but it sounded like a good solution. I felt a bit like the bionic woman, it was like they were going to re-build me!

That little uncertain niggle at the back of your mind ... are you sure? It said. I believed my niggle was much bigger than most. The more I listened to it the bigger it grew. Nicky's niggle ... it lived in the corner of the house, hidden from most everyday goings on but I thought it had a megaphone and audio system! Which allowed access to every room in the house,

Are you sure that's right? ... Are you good enough? ... Was it OK to do that? ... But what if?

Doubt and insecurity bellowing through the corridors of my mind hindering my life in every way possible. So, I tried to find the volume to turn the racket down. No niggle deserves such prominence in the house. Despite the niggles, I'd never been so sure of anything in my life, I knew surgery was the way to go for me even before I didn't have a choice.

Of course, there is always the choice to do nothing, but that was not an option for me. I wanted to live, and if necessary live with a bag, however, this mitrofanoff operation would give me an internal reservoir, this meant I would be continent, with nothing on the outside except my scar.

The consultants were happy that I would cope well with the difficulties during and after the operation, and I was a good candidate. After lengthy explanations of what was involved in my new plumbing, I gave my consent for them to book a date for my operation.

Chapter 3

Sleeping in the Midst of Battle

B e careful what you wish for, as I had gone from a person whose tears would flow so freely it annoyed me, to not being able to cry. So many times I'd just wanted to have a good cry and let it all out, but this just wasn't possible any more. *I had a problem with my eyes, I had severe dry eye syndrome and blepharitis, and they got extremely sore and irritated. To add to that, I physically couldn't cry. Even onions didn't make me cry any more and it had been like that for a few years. It had been a job getting the doctor's to believe me, as this was unusual even with my eye conditions.*

I couldn't cry at my daughter's wedding, the emotion was there and my nose would still run, but no more tears, it was utterly strange. She was so beautiful and the day was so lovely, how could I not cry?

Holding back the dry tears had become a thing for me then, as still it would be apparent by my facial expression that I was indeed upset. Sometimes I would cry in the shower, just to feel the water running down my face, and I could pretend I was normal again.

In the run up to my operation date, I had to do a lot of walking to try and get my fitness up, so I did as I was told.

I didn't hold back my emotions, I got upset at times, but I felt resolute in my attitude. I knew what was happening was for the best outcome, and would actually save my life, this is what I held onto.

In just six months, I had gone from seeing a small amount of blood in my pee, to staring a major operation in the face. This operation would involve:

- Removing my bladder, urethra, surrounding lymph nodes, uterus, ovaries and fallopian tubes.

- Harvesting some of my intestine and my appendix then constructing an internal reservoir with access via my tummy button.

When I found out the surgery included a hysterectomy, it was just sort of added on like a buy one get one free offer ... oh by the way we will be removing all this other stuff as well as your bladder. I knew they had to do it, those organs were in close proximity to my bladder and it could've spread.

The things that go through your mind at these times are hard to pin down, but I was already scared of going through the menopause, being 49 it was imminent. Then, I had to well and truly face it, along with everything else afterwards.

Aunt flow visited for the last time. Every month from the age of thirteen I had to endure her (well apart from when I had the kids). I wouldn't miss her, but I would miss being spoilt with chocolate, a hot-water bottle and rum.

The enormity of it all was blowing my mind, and of course, I questioned why this happened. I was relatively young, most people got bladder cancer later in years, and smoking was a big risk but I didn't smoke. I could've lived a healthier life, but I could've done a lot of things! The doctor's ended up just saying I was unlucky as nothing really stood out as a reason for me getting it. There are always exceptions, and I happened to be one of them.

Leading up to the date, I spent time shopping for little things for me to take to hospital, some new toiletries that were bright and cheery, new dressing gown (light weight as I though I would be hot), clothes that were stretchy and comfortable for after the op, and a nice pair of boots for when I felt better.

I visited town a few times, sat in coffee shops just reflecting on my situation. I knew I would feel pretty crap for quite some time afterwards so I planned ahead. I said to myself, "Nicky, you have to be careful or you may end up getting depressed after this".

A few days before my op, I was required to go to my local hospital. This was to get measured up for a stoma, just in case my mitrofanoff surgery failed for some reason and I would then wake up with a bag for life instead. The nurse basically drew a big X in the appropriate position on my tummy and covered it with a transparent plaster, so it didn't wash off before the day of surgery.

I thought about death a fair bit, I always had, but even more so then. Cancer has a way of showing you without a doubt, you are very mortal. I didn't fear it, but I wanted to have lived my life enough. It had crossed my mind that I might not wake up after the surgery, but I didn't dwell on it, I had a deep down feeling that I would be fine.

Ever since my mum died I thought I would die young and when I turned forty I had achieved the same age she was, and I looked on any more years as a bonus. My dad was in his fifties when he died, still cut short in my opinion. There was no cancer connection in the family as far as

I was aware.

Cancer was a sneaky thing and although I tried to think positive, now I'd had it, the thought was always there, one of my niggles. I guess death was always waiting for us, it was a sure thing in life. I felt I had annoyed him somewhat by delaying my demise for a bit. I always used my sense of humour when thinking about these issues, it was the best medicine for the mind.

I had spent a couple of years working as a carer in a Nursing Home, and it was inevitable that death was a fairly regular occurrence. Sometimes we had to prepare the dead, washing them and dressing them, and we would talk to them as if they were still alive. My colleague said to me when I first carried out that job with her, to make sure a window was open during that time for their spirit to fly away and avoid the Home becoming haunted. The Home was a big old building, it was like a maze of corridors, I certainly didn't want to risk it becoming haunted!

It was sad, getting to know these people and caring for them, but trying to keep a professional distance because you knew their time was short. If you got too close to people it was so hard.

I met some great people, staff and residents but I had to change this job, it was draining for me, and the shifts were so bad. I managed to get some part-time hours in the pharmacy, so I did both jobs for a couple of months, until I could get more hours at the pharmacy and quit the nursing home. It was a good move.

It was my last normal weekend, so Mick and I went out for a few drinks. More time for reflection on what was going to happen, and jokes about how soon I would be able to pee up a tree and write my name in the snow! (Mick said he'd have to take me up North in winter, as we never get enough snow round here).

I had continued to work through the weeks leading up to the operation, but I booked the Wednesday off, the day before I went in.

Again I went to town, and met Mick and we had a sort of "last supper", only it was lunch when Mick was on his break.

I felt nervous about it but at the same time wanted to get it over and done.

At the pre-op appointment a couple of weeks before, it was sweltering in the waiting room, we were slumped in our chairs, melting. We waited so long, then it turned out there was a mistake and I had been missed. The lady on reception was apologetic, and we didn't have to wait too much longer. The nurse I saw gave me six bottles of a pre-op drink. I was instructed to drink four bottles the night before and two first thing.

That night, I checked my bag had all I needed, and Mick had some crosswords etc. for his long wait, so everything was ready to go. I sat and drank the pre-op, it was very hard going, I didn't like the taste but I managed. Obviously, I couldn't eat after a certain time. I put my last post on Facebook and it was uplifting to read messages from friends, although I couldn't avoid getting a stress headache. An early night was needed as we had to be at the hospital for 7.30am, and it took nearly an hour to get there.

Early mornings aren't my thing, but I didn't have to worry about breakfast (only those drinks), and I thought soon I will be fast asleep for most of the day anyway. I went to the toilet noting that it would be the last time ever, I would go in that way.

Mick had taken me to the coast many times, for weekends and overnight stays during my uncertain times, he knew how to keep my mind occupied and distracted. I didn't mind getting up early to go away to the seaside!

The drive to the hospital went without a hitch. Once we got there we didn't have to wait long, and after talking to the anaesthetist, and various other people, I had to get changed in a gown and put on some very unflattering stockings, plus some non-slip socks. I was labelled on both wrists, all jewellery had to go so I gave Mick my ring for safe keeping, and he also had my phone.

So the time came, we had a hug and a kiss and said see you later. I wandered down the corridor with the nurse to the operating theatre, making nervous small talk.

I saw a lot of people in there, I recognised a few, and the anaesthetist asked me to sit on the edge of the table. He had to position an epidural in my back for when I woke up, this would make it easier for me to get moving after the op. Once he was done, I lay down and they confirmed with me who I was, and asked me what the operation was (although I was hoping they knew this already!), and they checked my labels quite a few times just to make sure it was me. They took my glasses and labelled them. I was attached to some machines, and the anaesthetists voice was the last thing I heard, then I fell asleep.

Chapter 4

Mr Mitrofanoffalus

My mouth was so dry, and opening my eyes, I looked at my hands and every thing around me, it was blurry so I asked the nurse to help me with my glasses. She had a friendly face, which I was glad to see. I had expected all of what I saw before me, but still I had a sinking feeling, followed by a relief that I was still alive. I asked if the surgery had gone according to plan, because I couldn't tell, and she said it had gone very well.

I had five tubes and containers attached to me, two on the left side for drainage, one in my belly button for urine and two on my right side also for urine. I could hear the usual hospital bleeping noises, there were a lot of gadgets around. I was told I had been thirteen hours in theatre, longer than the eight or nine that was expected.

The idea behind having three bags for the urine is for a couple of reasons, firstly having all these took the pressure off my new bladder, aiding it to heal properly, and secondly my bladder being made of intestine produced a lot of mucus which can block tubes, the more bags the less chance of blockage.

I used to work at a school for special needs kids, and then after that job I worked as a carer in a nursing home. I was used to seeing people with catheter bags, feeding tubes etc., people with sores that needed a lot of care and attention, and people dying from various things including cancer. I had seen a lot more than I wanted to, and I couldn't unsee it. I knew there were people worse off than me, people who didn't live to be very old, and the people who would say they had lived too long.

I asked for Mick and they said they would go and find him. The first 24 hours were in recovery, being watched closely. I was only allowed sips of water, and they tried to get me to drink this horrible thick shake drink, and that wasn't happening.

Mick had been waiting all that time while I was in theatre, he was shattered. He sat with me and I remember telling him to get some rest but he didn't, not until the nurse told him.

The epidural the anaesthetist had positioned in my spine turned out not to be as effective as I had been told, and not quite in the right position for the pain relief needed. It was supposed to block that area so I could move about without pain in the early days. They kept testing it with cubes of ice on my skin, some was numb, some was not so numb. I was told it must be having some effect or I would be screaming in agony, all I know is when I moved it was painful. I was told I could have extra pain relief if needed.

The physio's got me moving really soon, I had so many tubes and luggage but I managed it very slowly, onto a special chair they had brought in for me, and I actually felt comfortable in it and more relaxed, however; just two minutes later the nurse came in saying I had to get back in bed, so they could put a PICC line in! I couldn't believe it!

The nurse was really excited about me getting the PICC, she said it was great, they can then use it for intravenous antibiotics, nutrition and draw blood if needed. Seeing as I wasn't drinking those shakes and only sipping water, I guess that wasn't a bad idea. Once I had it installed I would be able to go down to the ward.

Like I said before, my mouth was so dry, I can't express how uncom-

fortable that makes a person, I was only allowed small sips of water, and those shake drinks were thick and just stuck in my mouth making it worse. My Mick being ever practical, bought me some lip balm, mango flavour. Something as simple as this, makes all the difference in these circumstances.

Two young men walked towards me wearing scrubs, and it took so long setting out everything for the PICC procedure, I was wondering what the heck they were going to do, but in fact once they started, it only took a few minutes! It went in through the side of my neck, but it didn't hurt.

When the PICC was in, there was talk of me going onto the ward and by the time I got to there it was late into the evening.

Hospital didn't really agree with my skin, I was allergic to the pillows (under the pillow case, they had a sort of plastic coating) and came out in a rash when they touched my skin. Also they gave me an antibiotic I turned out to be allergic to and another itchy rash broke out. My temperature kept on fluctuating, it was so hot, they gave me my own personal fan.

I slept most of the time in the early days. I didn't want to do anything else. I would see Mick sitting reading a book, and I'd doze off again, I knew he was there and that's what mattered. I felt looked after and had to put myself in their hands.

My consultant/surgeon came to see me on the ward the next day. She said I looked glamorous, and I laughed. She was very happy with how the operation went, despite how long it took, and she mentioned that my appendix was "cute", but it did the job.

I had a massive surgical wound which would need constant care, re-dressing every day until it healed. It wasn't an easy dressing either, my wound had holes which needed packing carefully, and it wasn't in a straight line, it went from above and round my belly button all the way down.

I was looked after very well in hospital, of course it was hard, I was expecting it to be. I had to go through it. I kept my sense of humour most of the time. The physio's were really tough, but they have to be to get people moving when they hurt, but I never saw that nice comfy chair again! I had to sit in that horrible bedside chair.

I had been told it's important to move as much as possible, of course this goes against the grain when all you want to do is sleep!

One morning, as they encourage you to do as much as you can, I was brought a bowl and flannel to wash with, and helped to the edge of the bed. The nurse went, she drew the curtains round and I sat. I was covered in an itchy rash, with tubes coming out every where, a cannula on each hand with what they call 'octopus' jangling each time I moved my hands, there were four tubes hanging out of each cannula (it amused me that they called it an 'octopus', Mick had said I had 'octopi' as I had two of them).

Well, my cheery persona was being tested that day. I looked around, what a state I was, and I felt so helpless. I had been trying to be upbeat for the nurse's sake but she found me broken when she came back.

That lovely lady helped me that day, she said, "how about a hair wash?"

I said "how?"

Off she went and got this cap, it goes on your head and you can wash your hair without getting soaked! My goodness I felt better, and again, it's the simple things that make a difference. By the time Mick came in to visit, I was much happier.

A few days in, I hadn't had much of an appetite but this day I was looking forward to my lunch, I had chosen something I really fancied.

The doctor's had other plans and wanted me to go for some scans, so I was ferried on my bed down all the corridors. It wasn't a pleasant time, moving off the bed to be scanned was very uncomfortable, anyway, when I got back, Mick was there which was nice but I felt very pee'd off with everything, I could smell the lunch that I was missing, then they told me I had to go back and have another scan; it was a hard day. Mick came with me that time. I knew all those things were necessary but I just wanted my lunch!

Mick visited every day, then one day I got a whole load of visitors, my three son's and my daughter and son in-law, it was a boost to see them all, but I was well knackered when they left.

Day and night they would come and take my blood pressure and temperature. They would also come and flush the urine bags I had. More mucus is produced when there are in dwelling catheters, and I had plenty of those. I was eight days in hospital and they took two of the bags away while I was there.

Sleeping at home I had a machine that mimicked the ocean waves to send me to sleep, or when I was in bed cosy and warm, I loved to listen to the rain outside and on the window. It would help to clear my mind and lull me to sleep,

I slept a lot during the day in hospital because I kept being woken up during the night, if it wasn't because they had to take my blood pressure etc. it was someone else on the ward pressing the button or a machine bleeping, usually it was my machine!

On the eighth day there was talk that I might be sent home, I managed a shower in the morning, although it wasn't easy by any stretch of the imagination.

They had to make sure I could cope being sent home, so the physio lady came to assess me. I had to put the non slip socks on, walk up and down the corridor outside the ward, and go up and down a flight of stairs. I was so determined to do this, I hobbled along slowly, I so wanted to go home. Thankfully I passed the tests so I had cleared that hurdle.

There had been another hurdle that I was told about but I had jumped over that one quite a few days before, when I tentatively did a number two. This would be important after any operation but as they had been fiddling around with my intestines, the dr's and I were happy my innards were working as they should.

As the day went on concerns were raised that my temperature was too high, and the nurses didn't think I would be sent home!

Time went on and at teatime I was tucking into some sandwiches, when my consultant came to see me. There were quite a few onlookers with him, the nurses who had obviously told him about my temperature. He said it was great to see me looking so well, and he thought it was time for me to go home, and I agreed, despite a bit of a temperature, which had been up and down all the time. I looked at the nurses who were a bit taken aback, and they now had to get all my paperwork and other stuff in order, plus show me how to look after the bags.

Two catheter bags were attached to my right side and another coming out of my bellybutton (this one I nicknamed Mr Mitrofanoffalus). I had to learn how to look after them, flushing them regularly. I would have to live with those three bags for six weeks, I had to wear those surgical stockings too, and I had to inject myself each evening as well.

They had to take out my PICC line, and the cannula's, sort out everything I needed to take home with me. Finally, I was in a wheelchair, and Mick wheeled me out, I was going home.

Chapter 5

Quest For Freedom

For me home means comfort, safety and family, my consultant knew that I would thrive better sleeping in my own bed and having my own routine. He said there comes a point where hospital had done it's job and to stay any longer could only cause problems for the patient. He made that call for me, and he knew what he was talking about.

I had a tough six weeks ahead of me, and I'm not going to lie, it was hard. Mentally, I had to try to keep myself stable, trying to look towards the light at end of the tunnel. Physically, it was uncomfortable more than painful but I had little energy so everything was such an effort.

I had one advantage though, my husband. He looked after me but more than that, he got me doing things and even taking me out. He kept reminding me this was for the short term.

I struggled out of the wheelchair and into the car, carefully arranging my tubes, and placing a cushion on my tummy to protect it from the seat belt. I noticed the car seemed to smell of Mick's sandals, not surprising as he said he had slept in the car that first night, plus all the journeying backward and forward for visiting.

I was a little anxious going home and having to deal with it all, I worried I wouldn't do it right.

We had already moved the bed round before the op, so that I was on the right side of the bed, to accommodate my bags and the accompanying night bags. Getting into my own bed, even though it was awkward, was still much more civilized, I slept well with no interruptions.

From the minute I was home, my rash started to clear up nicely, and each day a district nurse had to come and re-do my dressing, the wound would ooze, and it needed packing in places to help it close up properly. Some nurses did it better than others, but I remained so grateful for their help, and if it needed patching up I always had plenty of spare dressings.

My appetite was not much to speak of and as Mick had to go back to work he made me little meals each day that just needed heating up. It was more difficult for me without Mick, but in the early days my daughter would come in and help me depending on when her shifts were at work.

I had my routine, but by the Wednesday something went wrong, I was in pain and leaking through my belly button, I didn't understand what was going on because I had done the flushes how they said. When Mick came home, he rang the ward in advance, we had to go to Addenbrooke's, it was like labour pains.

Waiting to be seen I was pacing the floor, then sitting, then moving again, I was soaked and holding a towel to my stomach. Finally, help arrived and they attached a syringe to one of the catheter's and pulled back, they emptied quite a lot of mucus and pee, it had been blocked, despite me flushing. I was told how to take the mucus out with the syringe after that. I would never forget the pain and panic that I felt, I would never want to have that happen again. However, this incident showed my new bladder was strong and able to cope under pressure even at that early stage.

As the days went on I grew a bit more confident with my situation, Mick took me to visit work, and we popped out on a few other occasions, for a coffee and suchlike.

We'd always been great coffee consumers, our local coffee shop knew us as 'large americano and small skinny latte'. When I first met Mick it was for coffee, and we carried on the tradition over the years, meeting if I was off work and he had a break. For coffee and the seaside are probably the places we most liked to go, and preferably combining the two!

Back before the operation, when Mick and I were discussing things with the consultant, we mentioned that we had already booked a holiday to Scarborough, we always go in October. He saw no reason why we couldn't go, in fact he said it might be good for me. After the op, I did have my doubts, but thought we will just have to wait and see.

Four weeks post op, the district nurses entrusted my wound packing and dressing to my lovely nurse for the week … Mick!

Off we went to Scarborough for five nights to our usual hotel, urine bags and all. We went every year, so it was a home from home for us, and perfect for me to convalesce.

I was unable to attach all the urine bags to my legs, although I gave it a good try. Instead I had a shoulder bag that concealed my bags and tubes, which allowed me to potter about.

The case we took was full of dressings, sterile water, syringes, gloves etc., we were prepared for all eventualities and the rest. Nothing was going to keep us from the seaside.

Even if it was going to rain, it would never stop us enjoying our holidays, as long as we were dressed appropriately.

When the kids where very young, I would dress them in their wellies and macs and we would go out in the pouring rain just for fun, splashing in the puddles, it was better than staying in all day.

On the way, we stopped off to see a couple of friends who lived in Yorkshire, they also had a few chickens that I liked to go and see! (before I had chickens) We had a good catch up and lunch before heading off again to our final destination.

My appetite wasn't quite back to normal but I was doing ok, although two lots of antibiotics put a bit of a downer on it. One to take with food, and one without, and I wasn't able to have alcohol with them.

Each day we would take our time getting up, and Mick would change the dressing, he had watched the nurses and once he had that apron on he was like a pro.

He had me in stitches when he decided to wear little else one morning, just the apron and gloves! Then he wondered why I was giggling and not keeping still!

After a couple of days at the coast, the sea air was doing me the world of good. My appetite was returning, due to a spicy platter we shared one evening at the hotel. We took taxi's a lot, and I rested when I needed to. Mick's sister and her husband had been staying near Robin Hood's Bay, so we took the opportunity to meet up at a little cafe half way. It wasn't a normal holiday, but it was still good.

Going to the Sea Life Centre has always been a joy of mine, and my eagerness to go was still there on this trip to Scarborough. However, It didn't turn out how I had planned; the place was crowded and kids were running around, I felt so vulnerable with my bag over my shoulder, hiding the secret of my three urine bags. I imagined being bumped into or my bag being pulled from my shoulder, the thought of it made me panic. We had to leave and when I got out and sat in the car I was disappointed with myself. Disappointed I had let it get to me like that, disappointed I hadn't been able to enjoy looking at the fish like I normally would.

My dream job was to work at the Sea Life Centre, in the gift shop. No stress, and living by the sea. One day maybe.

After we returned home, the district nurse recruited Mick to carry on changing my dressings in-between times (as he was good at it) so the nurses' didn't have to come in everyday.

Each day when my wound was being re-dressed, they would pack parts of it with a special ribbon, it would ensure the wound healed from the bottom, up. Most mornings I would wake up and look down at my tummy and there it was ... I called it 'the slug', it was like it had crawled out in the night. This piece of ribbon that had soaked up the slime that came from my wound and then oozed itself out as I moved in bed.

I reached the six week mark, this meant I could take those horrible stockings off for the last time. I had only been allowed to take them off for about half and hour a day, and I had to wear them at night as well. Oh the satisfaction of throwing them in the bin!

All the little disposable syringes that I'd jabbed my self with every night were used up. Now things were getting interesting, the time had nearly come, and I eagerly awaited to go back to the hospital.

At around seven weeks post op, I had to go back to hospital for a scan and we didn't think we would be there that long, but when the results came back good, I was instructed to go to the ward to have one bag removed. A few days later we went back and they removed another, then I had to go in for an overnight stay before they removed my mitrofanoff bag.

My consultant/surgeon had to be called as the nurse was having trouble taking out my Mr Mitrofanoffalus catheter bag (they just wanted to replace it, and see how it was). I lay there and the nurse deflated the little balloon that keeps the catheter from coming out, put a bit of lube in my tummy button and pulled carefully, there was some resistance, she tried a few times but she could see it was uncomfortable for me.

We waited, and in she came in her scrubs, this lady exuded confidence and to say she had a formidable presence about her, was an understatement. After the nurse explained to her the problem, she got to work making sure the little balloon inside was indeed deflated then putting a whole load of lube in my tummy button. Twizzling the catheter and moving it up and down, then all of a sudden she pulled and popped it out! Oh, I felt it! ... I yelled at her "I knew you'd do that!!"

and as she pointed and smiled at the nurse, she replied "that's cuz I'm more of a bitch than she is!"

All of us had to laugh and I was glad she had managed to pull it out! They could then replace the catheter and attach a new bag.

Removing the first bag attached to my side was intensely painful! though it was over quickly. So, when I had to go in and have the second one removed, I took pain killers in advance hoping they would help ... they didn't and it was still agony! I was glad it was over quickly and it was worth it to gain my freedom.

Going back into hospital they removed my final bag with the catheter going into my belly button. For a brief few hours, I was free! And the specialist nurse taught me how to catheterise my mitrofanoff with these really long catheters, which would become my new best friends for the rest of my life.

As the bags were removed the feeling of being free from them was so wonderful. I knew the day would come when the tubes would be gone and I would feel comfortable once again. To be able to sleep on my side in the position I like once again.

Unfortunately, Mr Mitrofanoffalus decided not to play fair and after just three hours when I tried to catheterise, it wouldn't go in, the nurses tried, I changed position, nothing was working. I was panicking inside but the nurses remained calm, these were specialist nurses and they had dealt with this before.

I ended up having a procedure where they took me to radiology and they could look on a screen while passing a catheter into my pouch (internal reservoir). They had to put a very thin one in first and then increase the size. It was a tad uncomfortable, my tummy really ached afterwards and I had to have pain killers. The doctor left a catheter in with a tap on the end of it so I could empty the urine with that, rather than it going into a bag.

After the procedure the doctor didn't turn the tap off for me to move from the bench to the bed, and the urine leaked everywhere, I was soaked. I thought it best to clean up back at the ward, and the bed would need changing too. I just covered myself up on the bed while they took me back.

I had a bit of a moment back at the ward, when no one was there, I was upset as I had to go another two weeks with a tube in me, I was soaked and needed assistance and had to explain to the nurses what happened. Still, soon I was clean again and so was the bed.

I was gutted to be sent home that day, and know I had to return again in two weeks to try again. Freedom had been within my grasp, just for it to be taken away again so quickly.

The tap was much better than having a bag, I could just tuck it in my waist belt and it wasn't a problem. Yes, I was disappointed that I wasn't tube free, but the specialist nurse assured me that everything would be fine when I had it removed in two weeks. This was something that had happened before with similar patients.

I used to laugh and tell Mick it was like a little water pistol! And tell him I was quick on the draw. There was talk of making a holster out of a sock! but it never came to anything in the end.

I returned to hospital for them to remove my tap and catheter. This time all went well and I learned to catheterise through my belly button with no problems. I had to spend the night but went home later the next day.

After all my bags were removed the district nurse said because I was more mobile, I'd have to see nurse at my doctor's surgery for my dressing to be changed, so I said goodbye to the lovely nurses who had looked after my tummy at home.

Sleeping was so much better, so much comfier being able to move around with no tubes to hinder me. Before the operation I was getting up in the night for years, but since Mr Mitrofanoffalus came on the scene, no bladder calls!

Chapter 6

Wielding My Swords

On my school reports "quiet and conscientious" was often how my teachers described me and I believed them to be right. I had also been called "a dark horse" many times in my life, but not knowing the meaning of this, I didn't know whether to take it as a compliment or not. Having since found out, I agreed that maybe I was, but still wondered if they really meant I was a "mare with a shady disposition" or a "gloomy old nag"!

A quote from my face book profile; "Welcome to Nicky's world, a strange and yet fascinating place" of course I was referring to the world inside my mind more than my life in general. Although life and mind had been more in sync of late, I was mostly introverted, but with extrovert tendencies. The point was, the things I said were usually the tip of the iceberg compared to what I was actually thinking. What I found annoying was that in my mind I could make perfect sense, but when I tried to vocalise my thoughts, what came out? - utter crap! Nonsense of the highest order.

Brain and voice refused to connect, I'd hear rubbish being spouted and my mind was mumbling, oh no. It mattered once-upon-a-time but in that strange world that was Nicky, the older I got the more I didn't care, and maybe that's good.

It was expected that from then on I'd have to continue with appointments and scans at regular intervals for the rest of my life. The time between them would lengthen as long as all was well. My operation had been a success, there was a lot to be happy about and a lot to be thankful for.

I had been off work for three months and after Christmas my manager and I had discussed my return in January, part-time. It was a big step for me to think about going to work again.

That Christmas I actually managed to nearly cook the dinner, I felt it was quite an achievement, though I couldn't finish the job. Mick saw I was flagging and stepped in, he was much better at cooking than me anyway.

I missed Christmas' when the kids were young and I used to do a stocking for each of them. They would leave out a mince pie, a glass of milk and a carrot for Rudolph. My daughter wouldn't be able to sleep until she knew Father Christmas had been. In the morning, early as possible they would all be up, whispering on the landing, rustling paper from their stockings and comparing the treasure they had found. Waiting to be told they could go downstairs and see the presents under the tree.

The kids weren't kids any more, so it was different for everyone, time didn't stand still, even if we wanted it to. I always wanted it to snow, and it didn't have to be Christmas. I loved to watch it and stand out in it, covering up all the dirt and leaving a blanket, fresh and clean.

My surgical wound took ages to fully heal up, and I had to take a lot of antibiotics because of infections. I was left with a channel that went under the skin with a hole at each end. The nurses wanted it checked at the hospital at my next appointment.

I don't think the specialist nurse quite believed Mick when he said, "If you squirt the water in that hole with the syringe, it will spurt out the other hole, so watch out!" ... and what did he do?! Yes, he squirted it, and it nearly hit him in the eye!

There had been some very amusing moments, and I couldn't deny that I had laughed a heck of a lot. I had been at that appointment at the hospital for a check-up on how I was getting on with my mitrofanoff, but they wanted to check on why the wound was taking so long to heal. Funnily enough, after that it healed really quickly, we think the water dislodged something that had been delaying the healing and causing infections.

The nurse at the at the doctor's surgery was finally able to discharge me from her care. It had been at least four months and at last I would be able to have a bath instead of a shower!

At five months post op, I went back to thirty hours a week at work, I had been phased in with light duties and short shifts, but I felt ready to go back. It was important to find normality outside my comfort zone at home.

There were benefits to being in contact with the general public, people could be so funny at times, and we would have a little giggle. You'd get the nasty rude one's too, but most were pleasant. A lot of people didn't understand the workings of the pharmacy so they'd expect too much; if you said it would be twenty minutes, they'd stand there and stare at you, as if that was going to make it any faster!

Normally our pharmacy was open late and the last hour, from 10pm-11pm we had a night hatch. I managed to break the lock on it once, why was it always my shift? it was my shift when the fridge broke, it was my shift when the supermarket flooded because the roof collapsed due to a storm! (the pharmacy was inside the supermarket) all these incidents happened in my first year. On my first day, I pulled a shelf out and all the medications fell like a waterfall, I was very embarrassed. My manager said "Oh, nobody has ever done that before!". I used to have nightmares about the job. I did a lot of late nights and was responsible for locking up. I'm sure my checking routine rivalled that of Fort Knox!

I'd been getting on fine using the catheters, and I was in a routine of doing it four times a day. I found out one day that if I tensed my stomach muscles the pee flowed faster, and that was quite exciting, but no one told me that sneezing while you are mid flow had drastic results! I had a new understanding for the way men had to stand and pee, I know now why it could spray everywhere sometimes, and how annoying that could be; but there were no excuses for not cleaning it up!

My catheters were 40cm's in length and they were self lubricating. I obviously had to be careful, washing my hands before and after (or using hand sanitiser). I ordered them through a company who requested a prescription from my Dr, and then sent them to me directly. Each box had 60 in, and I would usually order 4-6 boxes at a time, then I knew I had enough for a few months, plus extras in case I had problems catheterising.

I would pretend they were swords and say "on guard!" while wielding one in front of Mick. (not while I was using it, I might add!)

I had to think of ways to carry my catheters with me all the time, it wasn't something I could do without, if I didn't have them I couldn't go to the toilet and that's serious. I got some little pouch bags and I kept some at work, in the car and in my handbag for every time I went out. I had to make sure I thought every time, making sure I had at least two with me, it was no good me forgetting or I'd have to go home.

I felt I was doing well with my body being thrust headlong into the menopause. I had mild hot flushes, anxiety was a worse thing for me and I had problems with brain fog at times which was so frustrating. It's not something you need when you are trying to advise a customer on their health issues

I know a lot of women suffer much worse, and this is just my experi-

ence, in my unique place in life. Again, I had an advantage, a man who could understand and spoil me at the right times, this helped a lot. I could be moody, but it really didn't last that long and according to Mick my brain fog was no different from normal!

Losing weight had always been difficult for me, and even more so after the op, I had to keep on plodding on with it though. The trouble was it was so slow going, it was driving me insane. We'd been eating so healthy, but still it seemed that wasn't enough to remove the bulk. I wanted to feel comfy in my own skin again and confident in myself, the daily struggle would just get to me. A whole week of it and I'd put ON a pound!

I was the sort of person who could live without sport and activities, I liked my comforts, and I didn't need to be doing something every minute of the day. I really didn't like that about myself but I couldn't change because that was who I was. Despite that, I did enjoy a good walk, and I liked dancing/aerobics, I was not a couch potato and when the kids were young I didn't have time to be. It just required effort on my part, to get motivated. I did have will power, but I had to really want to use it.

Chocolate at room temperature, the melt in my mouth texture. I loved a cup of coffee with chocolate, milk or plain. A special box of chocolates, ice cream or pancakes with chocolate sauce. Once I started, I couldn't stop. My body didn't love it though, I'd pile on the pounds at the mere smell of it, and it seemed to crave it! Best I stepped away from the chocolate and not have any.

Years ago I made a deal with my first father-in-law, he would give up sugar in his tea, and I would give up chocolate. It worked very well and lasted for nine months. I don't know if he went back to sugar in his tea or not, but I definitely went back to chocolate! but it made me realise I could do without such things, if I really wanted to, the trouble is I didn't really want to.

I'd had to be kind to myself those last few months, it could be a fine line between coping mentally and losing it completely.

For my birthday Mick got me some chickens. Three lovely fluffy chicks, they were bantams, smaller than the average chicken. I found them fascinating, I loved to watch them and tried to learn chicken language, you may laugh, but they were very sociable and communicative.

They would just decide at some point in the evening to all go to bed in the coop, even at that young age! I loved it so much! I watched them grow and no one was more excited when one of my chickens laid an egg! They were fabulous! And the egg tasted amazing!

As the chicks got older, I grew suspicious that I didn't have three hens in my flock, and that maybe one of them was a boy. I'd been told that the only way I would know, is when they lay an egg or crow!

Lets just say, my suspicions were correct when one morning my white chicken, Blondie, exercised his voice box. Only that wasn't the end of the story, as about a week later my silkie chicken, Cher, decided to get in on the morning chorus. These two cockerels had been brought up together, it was already decided between themselves that Cher was the more dominant of the two. Blondie learnt quickly to keep out of Cher's way first think in the mornings, and it was mostly only Cher's privilege to do the crowing. They were like brothers, and sometimes we would say Blondie is like Cher's side kick!

Of course, I had to get a couple more hens to join the flock, but I made sure they were hens!

I'd reached the half century and I didn't feel much different, even after everything, I'd realised there are many parts of me I could live without. If someone had told me what was going to happen during that past year, I wouldn't have believed them.

Living without my bladder was an everyday reminder to me, of all that had happened. I had mixed emotions about it, but that changed like the wind. Some days I was so glad and can see all the positives, having my Mr Mitrofanoffalus. Other days I was sad, seeing all the negatives, I was different to everyone else, and only a few people understood.

They had taken my womb like it didn't really matter, as I was old enough to be past needing it, I have my family, but still it was a part of being me, and I couldn't help having bad feelings about that.

My appendix had been just sitting there waiting to be used in a different way, it was my little hero, the 'dark horse' of my body. Who would've thought it would help save my life one day.

Eyes that couldn't produce tears any more. When I took my glasses off to wipe my eyes and found it dry, I missed the feeling of tears rolling down my cheeks, no matter how hard I tried I couldn't cry.

My innards had been shortened and rearranged to make my new bladder. I could feel the way it affected my body, I had to get used to the way foods were processed differently. I was down a few lymph nodes and my urethra was taken out.

All those things I was born with, but now I'd have to live without. I'd lived on without them in my new normal life.

I was happy to reach fifty and beyond. here I was, I was still me, still my personality tied up in the corridors of my mind.

The brain sounded more clinical than the mind … grey matter was it's internal make up, and the older I have become the more shades of grey I realise exist in my mind. Right or wrong issues used to be much clearer.

I thought that experience had made me this way. As there were always two sides to every story or even three or four.

Good and evil were not as clear, it was the way we all made our minds up about things and how we judged situations. The question 'but what if ...' when asked brings out a whole new perspective. I was slow to judge, we all did it but for some it came instantly and for others like myself, I liked to dwell on it for a while. The choices we make, shape our lives and we have to live with the consequences.

My grey matter had a lot to answer for if that was where my person-ality lived. I'd often wished I could change it, the complex person that I was is difficult to understand even for me ... and I was me! If only I could investigate me, I wonder what my findings would be. I dread to think! I'd always fancied the idea of being a psychiatrist, but maybe it's myself that needs to see one!

Chapter 7

Chicken Society

Sitting in the chairlift, both of us were terrified. As it pushed through the trees to the edge of the cliff, I could hardly breath. It was my idea, I wanted to go on it, knowing I would feel like that. I forced my eyes to open, to see the great expanse of the ocean, blue and beautiful.

In the distance we could see "the Needles", we would get much closer later on the boat, but we needed to get to the bottom of the cliff first.

Sometimes, life experiences make you a little braver, and this was one of those times. I don't like heights, I am scared on the bottom rung of a ladder.

It was a first time for us on the Isle of Wight, and we weren't disappointed. From the ferry over to the amazing view at our hotel, it was a smashing holiday.

I was still in my infancy regarding my new toileting issues, but I was used to making sure I had all my catheters to last the duration of the stay, plus my "emergency kit" which had lube and stuff for flushing, if I needed it.

At that point I was very positive about it all, I felt all was good and my situation wasn't stopping me doing any of the things that I loved. I could go on long walks, without worrying if there would be a loo along the way, as mine held more than my old bladder ever did. Plus, if I did need to go there was always the option of going behind a bush! Something I would try to avoid at all costs before, had become easy!

I had lost the urge to want to go to the toilet, so the way I knew, was when my tummy became a little uncomfortable, like I was over full. I would also keep an eye on the time, as I would normally empty every 4-6 hours in the day depending on how much I drank.

I can't say I missed that urge to go to the loo, I looked on that as a bonus, I mean you had to have some perks!

I reached my Mr Mitrofanoffalus anniversary, and I was happy to celebrate that day with a bottle of bubbly I'd saved from my birthday celebrations, as opposed to that disgusting pre-op drink I'd had the year before!

I was taking it all in my stride, I had no problems with it and when I went for my check-ups at Addenbrooke's, the scans and bloods were all good. It was almost like my new normal had become normal.

To all intents and purposes I looked "normal" and if someone didn't know about me, then I didn't need to tell them unless I wanted to. In some ways I liked that because I did like my privacy, but in other ways I felt rather alone in my plight. Either way, I didn't shout it from the roof tops, and if I did mention it, I noticed people really didn't want to know the ins and outs of my cancer, and how it was overcome. At times when I've wanted to share it, those people I thought would listen, did everything to change the subject.

I found some solace in chatting to people who had gone through similar things on the internet, I knew I wasn't alone. I had Mick to talk to, he understood it all, as he had gone through it with me.

Like struggles that go on in my mind, invisible to the outside world, I carried on in life.

I think it had lulled me into a false sense of security. The thing is you never know what's round the corner!

Then one day … I had leakage and couldn't get the catheter in!

I'd hadn't suffered much with leakage, but over a few days I had some incidents that were quite worrying to me. At work, it leaked and I had to go home, as I couldn't get the catheter in to empty it.

I was really struggling to get it in, and I got very stressed and worked up as this had never happened before. I changed position and tried again and again. I had to relax my self as I was tensing up. After nearly an hour, I'd managed it.

I tried to ring my specialist nurse at Addenbrooke's, he was hard to get hold of, and I was in a right state.

In desperation I called my doctor's surgery to try and get an appointment, making a fool of myself on the phone, trying to explain through my emotions. The receptionist sounded cold and uncaring, she didn't understand my situation. I had to call back up in the morning and then I got an appointment.

I was managing to get the catheter in eventually, but it was very tight. I thought I might have to go to Addenbrooke's.

I had been warned about going to the doctor with mitrofanoff problems, and even my local hospital, as not many have seen cases like mine, and some have never heard of it. If I definitely couldn't catheterise, I would have to go to A&E at Addenbrooke's. It would be a medical emergency.

The doctor was a locum I had never met, so I had to explain everything to him, it wasn't much use, but I did get a prescription for some more lube which was handy.

Finally, my specialist nurse got back to me, he wanted me to go in and see him that Friday which was a relief. Finally someone who knew what I was talking about!

It worked out well for Mick and I, as we had booked to go and see a pantomime at Gorleston-on-Sea on the Saturday. So we planned to go to the hospital and carry on to the seaside afterwards, staying for the weekend. Like I'd said before, not a lot can keep us away from the sea.

I explained to the specialist nurse my troubles, he said it would be best to keep a catheter in over the weekend with a tap on it, and then take it out on Monday, he said he would try and put a larger one into stretch it a bit. It's not unusual for this to happen apparently so, I agreed.

Unfortunately, it wasn't as simple as that, the mitrofanoff channel was so tight, he and I struggled to get a normal catheter in, let alone a larger one!

We were there for quite some time, and he couldn't get the one in that he wanted to, but I did end up with a catheter in, stuck with some tape to stop it falling out and a little pistol on the end.

Off we went to the seaside again, pistol and all! And having had this before, it was fine. I was happy not to have to struggle each time I needed the loo.

On the Monday, I took the catheter out and realised I was having some sort of allergic reaction to something, all round my mitrofanoff. The skin was so red and sore. I could catheterise fine but on the outside it was nasty.

After the surgery I'd had to get a medical bracelet as I was advised to do, and I wore it all the time, it had to be silver. My skin had a way of flaring up over things, it never used to when I was younger, but now I had to wear gold or silver, nothing else or I would suffer. So, it wasn't as Mick says, just an excuse because I have expensive taste!

I had quite a few weeks of health problems, what with the leaking, the soreness, and then it all scabbed over, it was pretty gross.

Not only that, I then had problems with my eyes. Going in to work one day I ended up not being able to see for half my shift because my eyes were so sore, and swelling up! It must of looked like I was winking at the customers!

It wasn't that I lived happily ever after, but that life continued to be a challenge.

I'd win my battles one at a time, with hopefully breathing space in-between to go to the coast with Mick. I had to get my priorities right!

Making memories and taking pictures. Living life, as it soon passes.

There was something special about a picture that had been painted. A snap shot in time but time had been spent on it, getting it right. Care and effort had been put in, attention to detail and a sense of pride in his work that was always is a pleasure to view. I'd expected good things and was not disappointed.

To be painted with my windmill meant a lot to me and that was thanks to Mick's dad. He would normally paint animals but he could turn his hand to most things. I could see his creative flare had been passed on down the generations.

My dad and my grandad used to take me to visit Stevington windmill when I was a child, I was fascinated by it and loved to explore it. In later years I'd re visited my old village which held so many memories for me. The cross, the church with it's holy well, and the tall rhubarb that grew there. The graves of my dad, grandma and grandad, all rest there.

Another year and another birthday was nearly upon me, I was hitting the ground running, despite tripping up every now and then, I was succeeding, carrying on in my little corner of the world.

Then the world itself was struggling, and they talked of a 'new normal' in their own way.

My freedom again was taken away, not just me but everyone, due to another deadly disease. Everything was uncertain.

I had a broody hen called Irtha. We weren't raising chicks so this behaviour was unfortunate. I had to get her out of the nest every now and then for her to have food and water, or she would stay there all day.

My other hen, Sandy, wanted to lay an egg, but I had shut the coop so Irtha didn't go back in. I noticed this as the other three chickens were gathered round Sandy, who was sitting in the pot which was laying on its side. Even when I went into the chicken run to do something, none of the chickens moved (most unusual). They were protecting her, as while she was laying an egg she was vulnerable.

As chickens, they knew a lot about protecting each other. Cher my cockerel, I believed, was brave enough to give his life to save his hens. Chickens are not really "chicken", they are just wary, as they should be, seeing as most things like the taste of them.

I had faced my giant, and the causeway had been destroyed. Like all other problems in my life I'd coped, with a down to earth attitude, a sense of humour and Mick. I wasn't brave, I just trusted others to help me.

I looked at the present and I was still there.

The future remained unwritten for me, and the world remained very strange.

Like in chicken society though, I hoped humans wouldn't forget how to watch out for those who were … 'laying an egg'.

The End

About The Author

Nicky Johnson

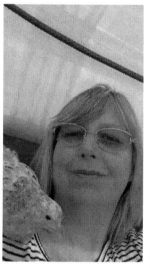 Born in Newport Pagnell, England, Nicky grew up in the neighbouring counties of Buckinhamshire, Northamptonshire and Bedfordshire. She is married to Michael Johnson and now lives near Bedford. Her first job was an office junior where she worked her way up to clerical assistant and assistant secretary. Bringing her four kids up at home until they were school age, she then worked at a special needs school for seven years before becoming a carer at a nursing home. Nicky now works at a local pharmacy. Having been inspired by her experiences and writing her memoirs for many years, "the parts of me I can live without" is her first book. She has also enjoyed writing poetry for many years. Nicky enjoys the company of her chickens and continues to learn chicken language.

Printed in Poland
by Amazon Fulfillment
Poland Sp. z o.o., Wrocław